Unplugged
Esacaping the Social Media Trap and Taking Your Life Back

Phillip Jason Taylor

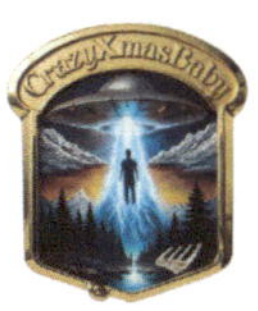

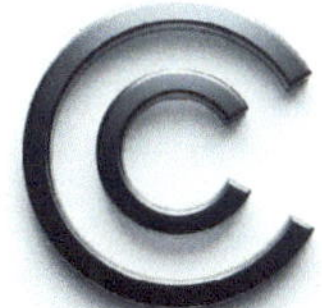

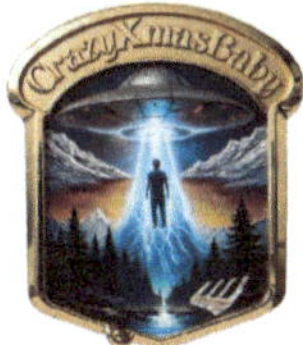

Learn More About CrazyXmasBaby Music

CONTENTS

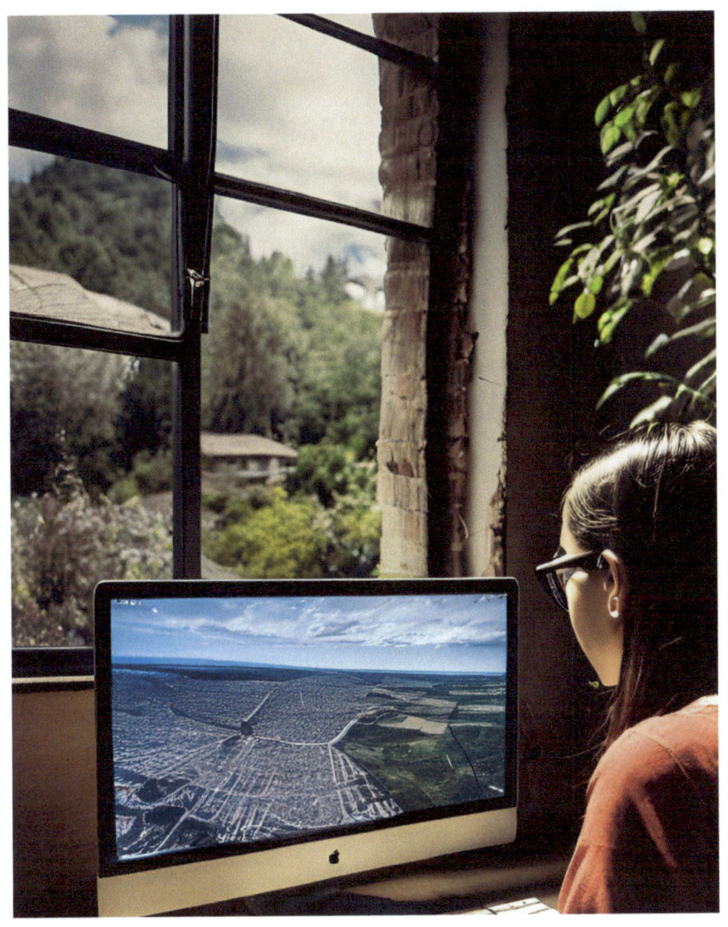

THE SOCIAL MEDIA TRAP

"Are you living your life, or are you just scrolling through someone else's?"

You've probably asked yourself this question before. If you haven't, it's time to. Social media was designed to connect us, but somewhere along the way, it has taken control of our lives. You log on for "just a minute," and before you know it, hours have disappeared—time you'll never get back. You're left feeling drained, anxious, and often worse about yourself than when you started. It feels like everyone else is living a life more interesting than yours. Spoiler alert: they aren't.

This book isn't just about quitting social media. It's about reclaiming your life.

In the digital age, we've been sold a lie that our worth is measured in likes, shares, and followers. We've been told that success is built online, that if you're not constantly promoting yourself on social media, you're irrelevant. But what if I told you the opposite is true? What if the key to real success, happiness, and fulfillment is found in disconnecting from the endless scroll?

The Real Problem

Let's get one thing straight: social media isn't inherently evil. It connects people, sparks creativity, and gives us access to endless information. But like anything powerful, it comes with a dark side. It's addictive. It preys on your need for validation and your fear of missing out. It makes you a slave to other people's approval and derails your ability to focus on what truly matters.

Here's a fact: social media is stealing your time, your energy, and —most importantly—your potential. And it's doing it under the guise of keeping you "connected."

But are you really connected? Or are you just distracted?

Why This Book?

I wrote this book because I saw too many people—myself included—getting lost in the digital abyss. We're more distracted than ever, more anxious, and more disconnected from our own lives. Somewhere along the way, we stopped living for ourselves and started living for the validation of others.

This book is for those who are ready to take control. It's for the creators, the entrepreneurs, the dreamers who want more out of life than a few seconds of digital attention. It's for those who feel like something is missing but can't quite figure out what. Spoiler: what's missing is your life—the one that's happening right now, beyond the screen.

What You Will Learn

In the pages that follow, I'll show you how to break free from the social media trap. We'll talk about:

- The Hidden Costs of Social Media: What it's really doing to your brain, your time, and your mental health.
- The Benefits of Quitting: From regaining your focus to unlocking your creativity, I'll show you the perks of unplugging.
- The Blueprint for Quitting: Whether you want to detox slowly or go cold turkey, I'll give you a step-by-step guide to take your life back.
- Building Real Connections: How to cultivate meaningful relationships and a thriving network without relying on likes and followers.
- Finding Success Beyond Social Media: How disconnecting can actually help you achieve more and be more successful in your personal and professional life.

A Bold Challenge

This isn't just a book; it's a challenge. I'm going to ask you to do something extreme: quit social media for 30 days. Before you roll your eyes, hear me out. It's not about giving it up forever—just long enough to see the difference it makes. If you're willing to take that leap, I promise you'll experience something most people in the digital age never will: real freedom.

By the end of this book, you'll have the tools to not only quit social media but to reclaim your time, energy, and potential. You'll be equipped to focus on the things that truly matter—your goals, your relationships, your passions.

This isn't about being a digital hermit; it's about becoming wildly successful in a world that's constantly pulling you in a hundred directions. If you're ready to stop scrolling and start living, then you're in the right place.

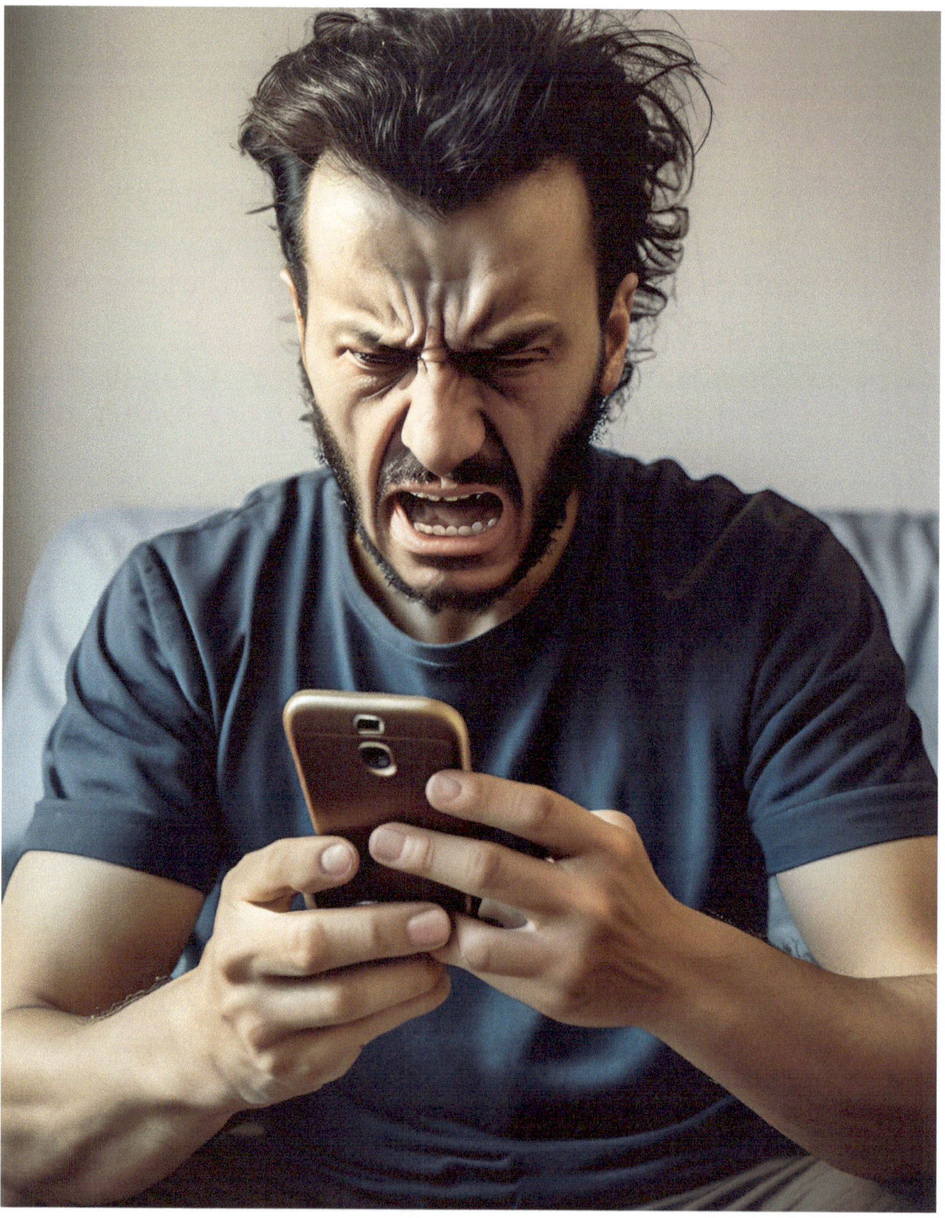

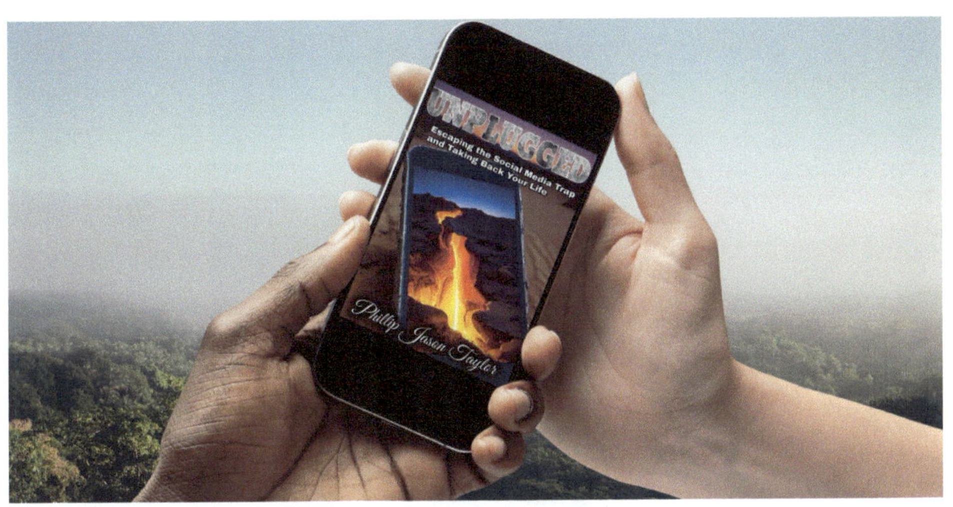

THE SOCIAL MEDIA TRAP

How Did We Get Here?

Take a moment and think about the last time you picked up your phone. Was it just out of habit? Maybe you planned to check something quickly, but before you knew it, you were scrolling, liking, and mindlessly consuming content. Does this sound familiar?

You're not alone. Social media has become the fabric of modern life—woven into everything we do. What started as a fun way to connect with friends and share moments has turned into a full-time distraction. The line between life online and real life has blurred, and for many of us, that line disappeared a long time ago.

So, how did we get here? How did platforms meant to connect us become the very thing pulling us apart from our true selves?

The answer is simple: social media platforms were designed to be addictive.

The Science Of Addiction

Have you ever noticed how it feels when you get a new notification? That tiny dopamine hit when you see that someone liked your post or commented on a photo? That little rush is no accident. Social media platforms are carefully engineered to keep you coming back for more, using the same psychological principles that drive addiction.

Here's how it works:

- Variable Rewards: Social media uses the same reward system that keeps people playing slot machines. Every time you scroll or refresh, you don't know what you're going to get. Maybe someone liked your photo. Maybe there's a new viral meme. It's this unpredictability that keeps you hooked.
- FOMO (Fear of Missing Out): Social platforms thrive on your fear of being left out. They know that if they keep you plugged in, they can exploit your need to know what's happening in your friends' lives, your industry, or the world.
- The Feedback Loop: Likes, shares, and comments are forms of digital validation, creating a loop of craving and satisfaction. The more you engage, the more validation you seek, and so the cycle repeats.

These platforms aren't just apps—they're machines designed to capture and monetize your attention. And here's the scary part: it's working.

The True Cost Of Social Media

Most people don't realize how much time and mental energy social media consumes. On average, people spend 2 hours and 31 minutes per day on social platforms. That's
over 900 hours a year—the equivalent of nearly 38 full days of

your life spent scrolling.

But the cost isn't just measured in hours; it's measured in lost potential. Social media pulls you away from what really matters—your goals, your productivity, your creativity, and even your happiness.

Let's break it down:

- Time Wasted: Imagine what you could do with an extra 900 hours a year. You could write a book, launch a business, learn a new skill, or finally pursue that passion project you've been putting off. Social media doesn't just steal your time; it steals your future.

- Productivity Killed: It's not just about the hours spent scrolling. Studies show that even brief distractions—like checking your phone for notifications—can derail your focus for up to 23 minutes. Social media makes it nearly impossible to get into a state of deep work, where real progress happens.

- Mental Health Crisis: Numerous studies have linked heavy social media use to increased rates of anxiety, depression, and loneliness. The endless comparison to other people's curated lives leaves you feeling inadequate. You're constantly bombarded with images of perfection, success, and happiness—none of which are real, but all of which make you feel worse about your own life.

The Illusion Of Connection

Social media promised to make us more connected than ever before, but has it really? Sure, your "friends" with hundreds, maybe thousands of people, but how many of those relationships are genuine? How many of those interactions bring you real joy, real fulfillment, or real support?

In reality, social media often makes us feel more disconnected, not less. It's easy to forget that behind every post, every filtered selfie, and every update is a person struggling with the same insecurities and doubts as you. But you don't see that. You see the highlight reel, the polished moments designed to show only the best parts of life.

Meanwhile, real human connection—the kind that happens face-to-face, or even through a heartfelt phone call—gets lost in the noise.

How Social Media Sabotages Your Success

If you're serious about achieving something big—whether it's starting a business, writing a book, or mastering a new skill—you need focus, time, and energy. But social media is constantly pulling you in the opposite direction.

Here's how it derails your success:

1. Distraction: Social media constantly interrupts your flow. You can't make real progress on anything if you're checking your phone every few minutes.

2. False Productivity: Many people convince themselves that social media is "work"—networking, promoting their brand, staying updated. But scrolling through feeds and obsessing over likes isn't the same as actual, productive work. It's busy work that doesn't move the needle on your real goals.

3. Mental Drain: Each time you engage with social media, you use mental energy—whether it's deciding what to post, reacting to someone else's content, or just consuming endless updates. This constant mental load leaves you too tired to focus on what truly matters.

4. Comparison Kills Motivation: Social media gives you a

front-row seat to everyone else's highlight reel. It's hard to stay motivated when you're constantly comparing your life to an idealized version of someone else's. Instead of feeling inspired, you feel discouraged.

Breaking Free From The Trap

Now that you understand how deeply social media is sabotaging your success, it's time to take action. In the next chapters, we're going to dive into the benefits of quitting and the steps you can take to regain control of your life.

Here's the truth: you don't need social media to be successful. In fact, without it, you'll have the time, energy, and focus to achieve more than you ever thought possible. It's time to break free from the trap and unlock your full potential.

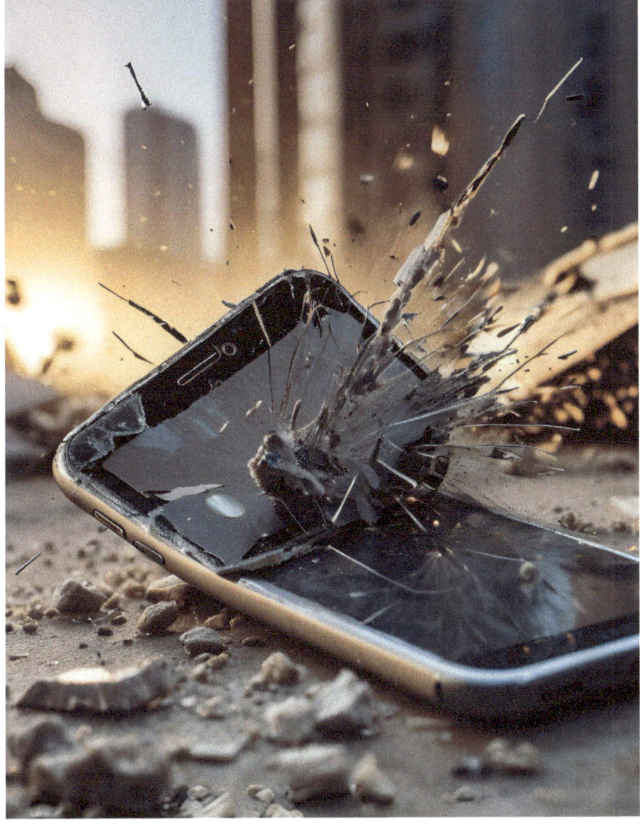

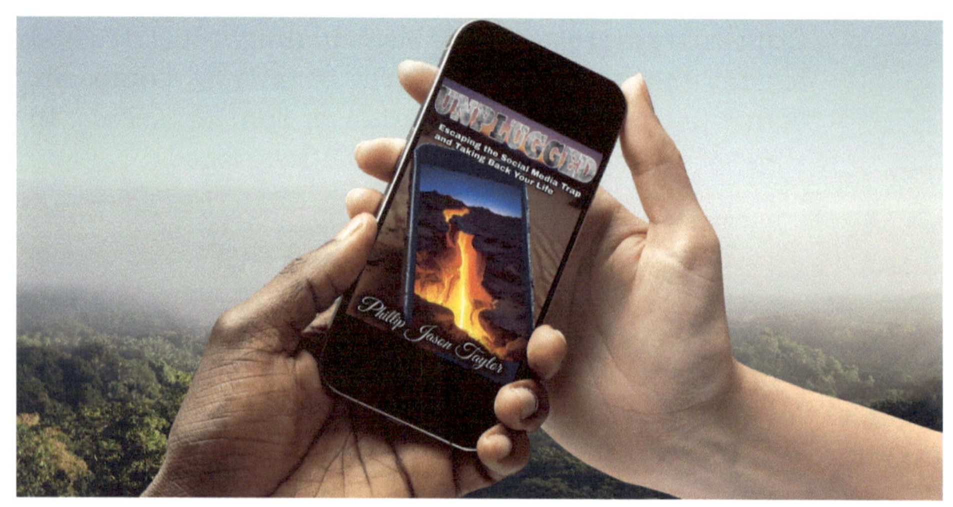

THE COST OF ONLINE VALIDATION

Welcome To The Popularity Contest

Here's a fun fact: your self-worth is now measured in likes, shares, and comments. Congratulations, you're officially a contestant in the world's most depressing popularity contest! Whether you realize it or not, every time you post a picture, share a tweet, or upload a status, you're essentially raising a digital hand and shouting, "Please, somebody, validate me!"

And, if no one does? Well, then you must be a failure, right? You didn't get enough likes, so obviously, the rest of the world is living more glamorous, fulfilling lives while you… well, you might as well not exist.

Except here's the thing: likes don't matter. But they sure do make you feel like they do, don't they?

The Dopamine Feedback Loop (A.k.a. The Digital Drug)

Let's be honest—social media is designed to feel like a slot machine, except instead of quarters, you're throwing in your mental health, your time, and, occasionally, your dignity. You hit the refresh button, hoping for that hit of dopamine that comes when someone (anyone, please!) engages with your post. And oh, the sweet, sweet satisfaction when they do.

But guess what? That little rush you feel? Yeah, it's not real. It's as temporary as the TikTok trends you were too late to jump on. Social media engineers know exactly how to keep you coming back for more, feeding you crumbs of validation so you stay hungry enough to keep chasing that high.

Congratulations! You're hooked. But at least you're in good company—billions of people are doing the exact same thing.

Let's Talk About The Illusion Of Success

So, you've got 10,000 followers on Instagram, 50,000 views on your latest TikTok, and a solid streak of Snapchats going with that one person you don't even like. You must be killing it, right? Wrong. You're not killing it. Social media success is an illusion—one that convinces you that follower count equals value.

Here's a little secret: no one cares about your follower count. Really, no one. The people who do care are the same ones refreshing their own feeds, obsessing over whether or not their lunch photo got enough engagement. It's a sad little loop of people trying to one-up each other in a game where the prize is... nothing.

Seriously. What exactly are you winning? A shiny blue checkmark next to your name that tells the world you've successfully wasted hours of your life curating a digital persona? Bravo.

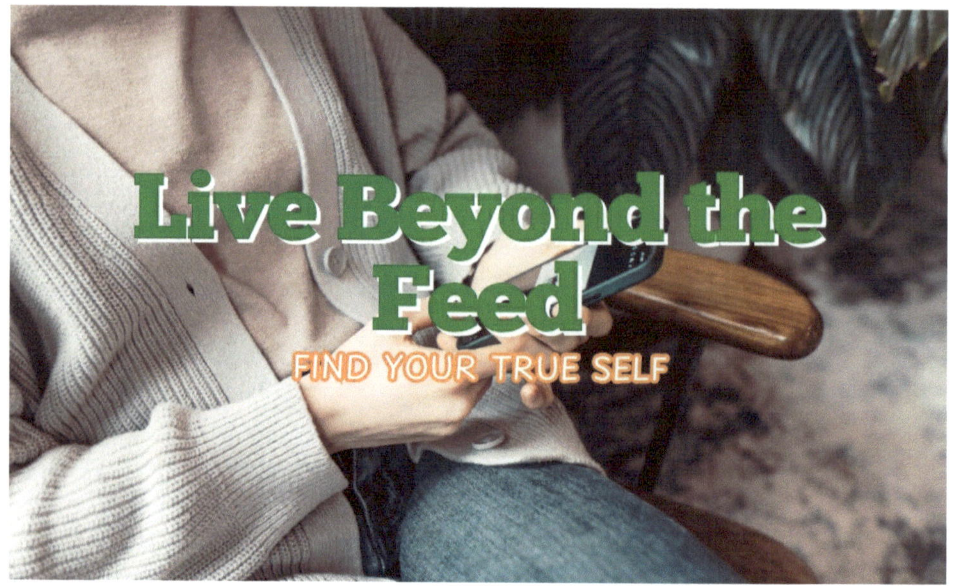

Chasing Likes: The Modern-Day Hunger Games

Every time you post something online, it's like entering yourself in the Hunger Games of social validation. You put yourself out there, waiting for the notifications to roll in, hoping your photo will somehow make it to the Capitol (or at least get a few dozen likes). And when it doesn't? Cue the self-doubt. The internal monologue that goes something like: "Am I boring? Why does nobody care? Maybe I should delete this post before anyone notices how little attention it got."

Sound familiar? That's because social media thrives on one thing: your insecurities. And boy, does it exploit them beautifully.

The truth is, likes are the cheapest form of validation. They're hollow, meaningless taps on a screen that ultimately don't reflect anything about you or your worth. But we still chase them because we've been conditioned to. We've bought into the lie that more likes, more followers, and more shares mean we're more successful, more interesting, or just more... important.

The Followers vs. Friends Dilemma

Ah, followers. The more you have, the more important you must be, right? Wrong again. Let's be clear: the number of followers you have is in no way a reflection of the number of people who actually give a damn about you. In fact, most of your followers wouldn't even notice if you disappeared off the face of the Earth—or, more realistically, just stopped posting.

You've probably heard the phrase "friends in real life." You know, the people who you could actually call up in an emergency, or who know more about you than what you ate for dinner last night. Yeah, those are the relationships that matter. Not the faceless followers who only engage with your content because it happened to show up on their feed while they were bored.

Real friends don't care about how perfectly curated your Instagram feed is, or whether your Facebook status got a dozen "likes." They care about actual, meaningful connection—something social media is severely lacking.

Replacing The Need For Validation

Okay, so now you know that chasing likes and followers is a waste of time (and energy, and self-esteem). But how do you stop caring about that little dopamine hit every time someone taps on your post?

Here's the tough love: you replace social media validation with real validation—the kind that comes from within. Yeah, I know, it sounds like something you'd hear in a cheesy self-help book, but hear me out.

The next time you post something, ask yourself why you're doing it. Is it because you genuinely want to share something meaningful? Or is it because you're hoping to get that quick hit of approval from people you barely know? If it's the latter, consider stepping back. Better yet, don't post at all.

**Instead, focus on building your self-worth
from things that actually matter:**

- Real accomplishments: Something you can look at and say, "I did that," instead of "I got 100 likes."
- Genuine connections: You know, those people who don't need to see your filtered selfies to care about you.
- Personal growth: Maybe learn a new skill or challenge yourself in a way that doesn't involve scrolling through someone else's highlight reel.

The Hard Truth: Nobody Really Cares

Here's the brutal truth that social media doesn't want you to know: nobody really cares. Not about your posts, not about your followers, not about your likes. And once you realize that, you're free.

Free from the pressure to always be "on." Free from the anxiety that comes from constantly comparing yourself to others. Free to live your life on your terms, not based on how many heart emojis you collect.

So, stop chasing validation from strangers online. You don't need it. What you need is to stop looking for approval in a place where it doesn't exist.

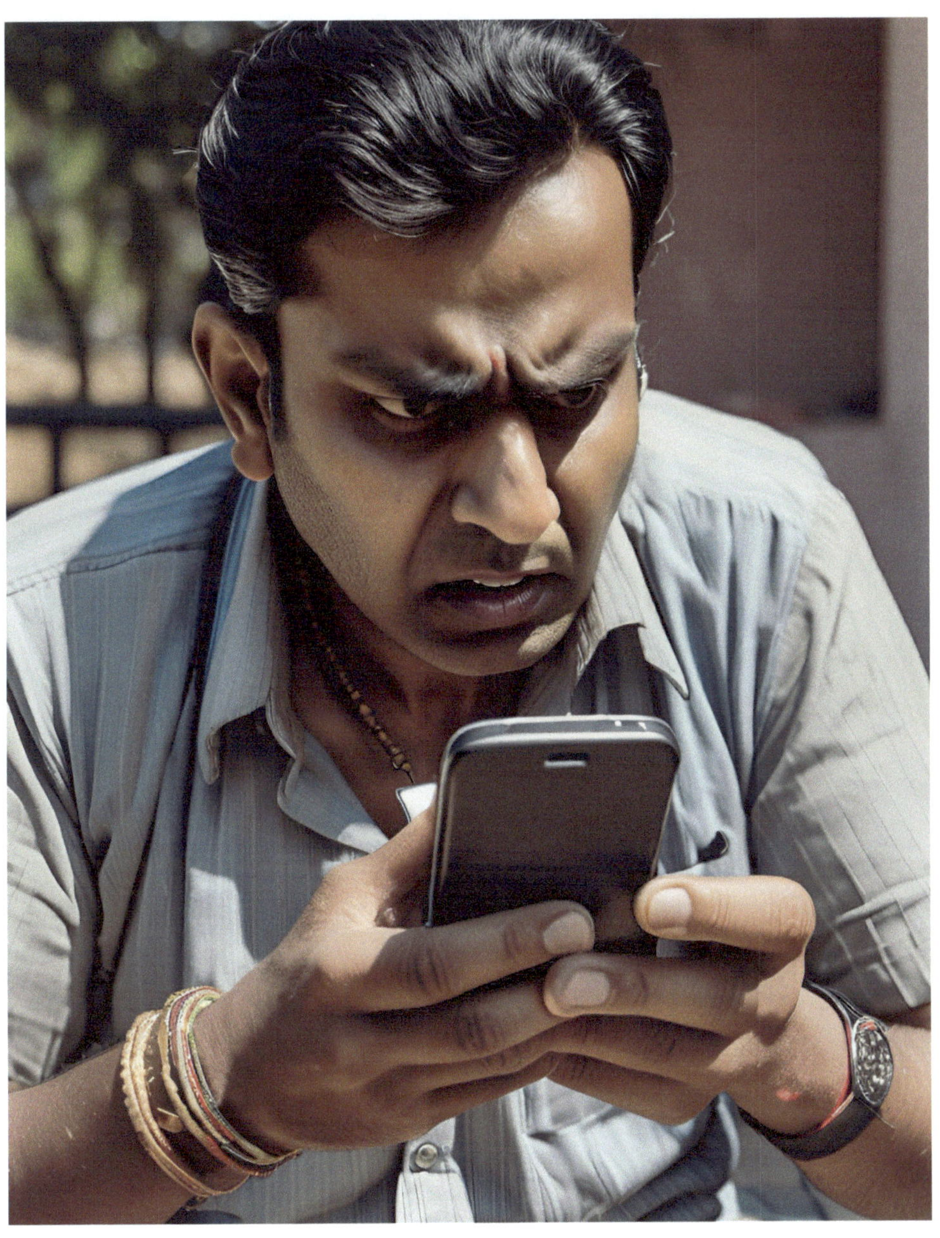

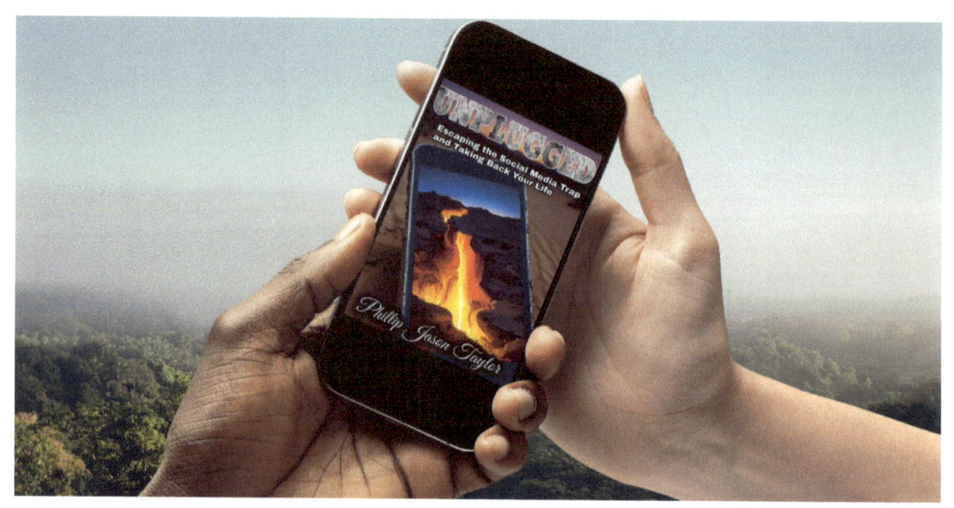

THE ILLUSION OF CONNECTION

Friendship: It's Not A Number

Ah, friendships in the digital age. Remember when "being friends" meant actually knowing someone, maybe having a few laughs together, or even, heaven forbid, sharing a meal? Now, it means having a little profile icon with a couple of hundred —or thousands—of other little profile icons. That's right, your "friends" are now measured by numbers, not actual human interaction.

The truth? These digital connections are about as meaningful as a five-minute soap opera plot twist. Sure, it's nice to see someone's vacation photos or random musings, but does it really count as a relationship? Spoiler alert: No, it doesn't.

The Faux Friendship Parade

Let's talk about those "friends" who like your posts, comment on your status, and tag you in memes. Do they know your middle name? Can they tell you your favorite color? Do they even know what you're passionate about? If you answered no to any of those questions, guess what? They're not real friends. They're digital acquaintances at best.

Here's a fun exercise: try calling one of these "friends" when you need help. I'm talking about a real, actual phone call, not a quick text or an emoji. See how many actually pick up. Go ahead, I'll wait. The results might be eye-opening.

The Real Value of Face-to-Face Interaction

So, you've got hundreds of "friends" on social media, but how many of them would actually show up for you in real life? True connections are built on real-life interactions—those awkward hugs, those long conversations over coffee, and yes, even the dreaded small talk. It's those moments of genuine human contact that create lasting bonds.

Let's be clear: there's no substitute for face-to-face interaction. Zoom calls and DMs might keep you in touch, but they're not the same as sharing space and energy with someone. There's something profoundly different about seeing a person's facial expressions, hearing their voice, and feeling their presence. Social media can't replicate that.

The Comparison Game

Social media is the ultimate comparison trap. Every time you log in, you're bombarded with images of everyone else's "perfect" lives. That couple in Bali? They've been married for three years. That guy with the new sports car? He's been working his ass off for it. And you? Well, you're probably stuck scrolling through these highlight reels and feeling like your own life is dull by comparison.

But guess what? That comparison is based on a lie. Social media is a curated version of reality, showing only the best parts of people's lives. It's like a movie trailer where you only see the dramatic, exciting scenes—leaving out the mundane, everyday stuff. You're not seeing the full picture. You're seeing the glamorous edited version.

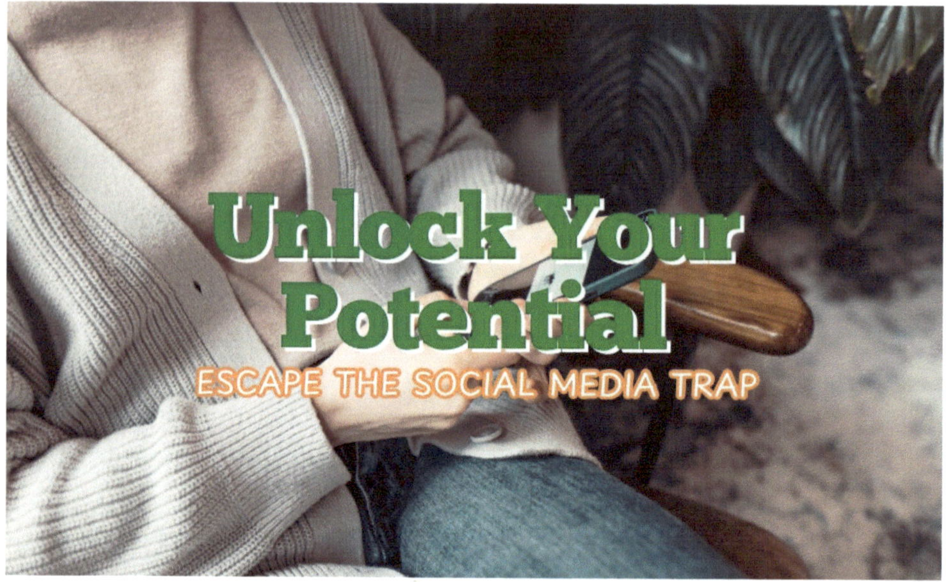

Why Social Media Connection Is Shallow

Let's face it—social media connection is as deep as a kiddie pool. You might have a lot of "friends," but how many of them are genuinely invested in your life? Social media connections are often shallow and fleeting. They're driven by algorithms and trends, not by real emotional bonds.

When you post something online, how much of it is really about sharing something meaningful and how much is about fishing for likes and comments? That's not connection—that's performance. And performance doesn't build real friendships.

The Freedom Of Real Relationships

Imagine this: no more worrying about crafting the perfect post, no more fretting over why that person didn't like your photo, and no more anxiety about whether you're "keeping up" with everyone else. Sounds blissful, right? That's what happens when you focus on real relationships instead of digital ones.

When you let go of the online connection game, you free yourself to build deeper, more meaningful relationships. Relationships where you actually know and care about each other, where you support each other's dreams, and where you share real experiences—offline. It's where genuine connection happens, and it's where you'll find true fulfillment.

The Secret To Building Real Connections

Here's a shocker: you build real connections by putting down your phone and actually talking to people. Go out, engage in activities you enjoy, join clubs, volunteer, or just strike up a conversation with someone new. Invest time and energy into relationships that matter, and you'll find that the superficial "likes" and "follows" fade into irrelevance.

Remember, the best friendships aren't measured by how many people know your name—they're measured by how many people genuinely care about you and are there for you when you need them. And that's something social media can't offer.

Now we'll explore the magical world of getting back your time and focus. Because once you drop the façade of online connection, you'll find yourself with more time for the things that truly matter.

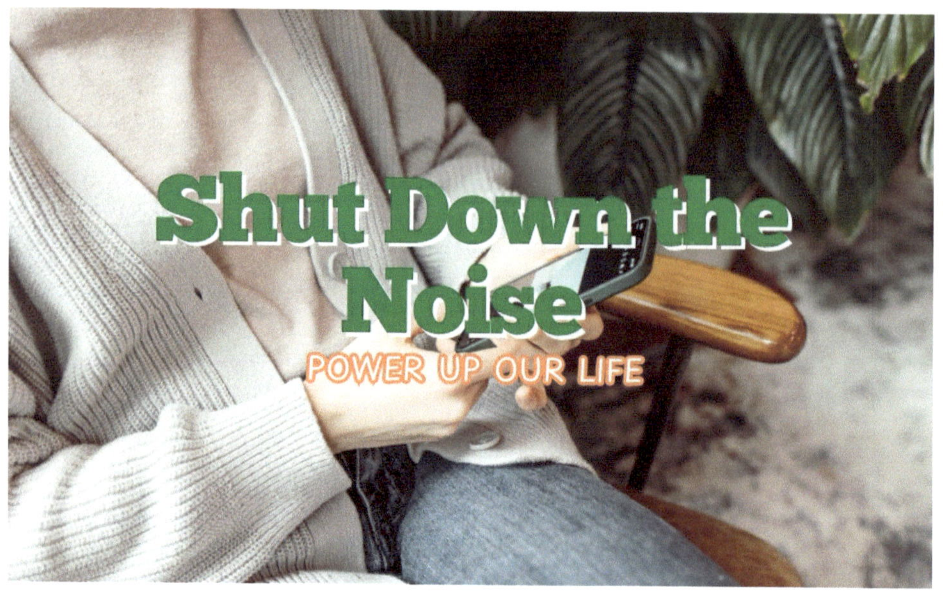

Shut Down the Noise
POWER UP OUR LIFE

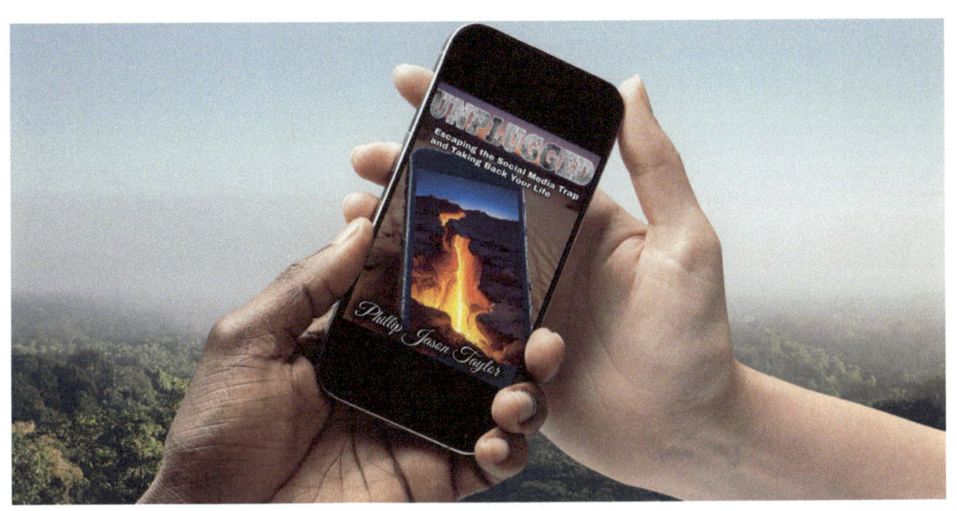

RECLAIMING YOUR TIME AND FOCUS

The Art Of Doing Nothing (And Loving It)

So you've decided to step away from social media. Congratulations! You've just taken the first step towards rediscovering what it means to be truly productive—and not just in the digital sense. Now, let's talk about one of the most underrated skills in our hyper-connected world: the art of doing absolutely nothing.

Yes, you read that right. Doing nothing isn't about being lazy; it's about giving yourself the space to think, create, and just be. Without the constant barrage of notifications and the pressure to stay engaged, you'll find yourself with an abundance of time. And with that time, you can actually start enjoying life instead of just documenting it.

The Time Sinkhole

Ever wondered where all your time went? You're not alone. Social media is a black hole that sucks in your hours, leaving you wondering why you haven't accomplished anything meaningful. But guess what? When you stop scrolling, you're left with a precious resource: time.

Think about it. If you spend 2 hours a day on social media, that's 730 hours a year. Imagine what you could do with that time:

- Write that book you've been putting off.
- Take a class and learn a new skill.
- Finally finish that DIY project you've started.
- Spend more quality time with friends and family.

The list is endless. And the best part? You're not wasting your time on fleeting digital interactions. You're investing it in things that matter.

Focus: The Forgotten Superpower

In our digital age, focus is like an endangered species. Social media is designed to fragment your attention into tiny, manageable bites. You can't focus on one thing for too long before the next notification pings you back into a distracted frenzy. But when you quit social media, you regain a superpower: the ability to concentrate.

Here's how it works: when you're not constantly interrupted, your brain has the chance to enter a state of deep focus. This means you can work on projects for extended periods without being derailed by digital distractions. You can dive into complex tasks, think creatively, and make real progress.

Imagine being able to sit down and work on something for an uninterrupted hour. What could you accomplish? Probably a lot more than you do while juggling social media interruptions.

Rediscovering Real Passions

Without the constant pressure to curate your online persona, you have the freedom to rediscover your real passions. Remember those hobbies and interests you used to have before social media took over? Now's the perfect time to revisit them.

Here's a wild idea: instead of spending your free time checking out what everyone else is doing, why not spend it doing what you love? Maybe it's painting, cooking, hiking, or even just reading a book. These activities not only bring you joy but also help you reconnect with yourself.

The Joy Of Genuine Experiences

When you stop living through a screen, you start experiencing life in the moment. You're not worried about capturing the perfect Instagram photo or crafting the most witty tweet. Instead, you're living fully in each experience.

Think about it: when was the last time you went to a concert, enjoyed a meal, or had a conversation without trying to document it for your followers? When you're not preoccupied with how things look online, you're free to savor the real moments. And those moments? They're often more fulfilling than any digital validation you could get.

Building Real Skills

Social media might give you the illusion of being productive, but it's not the best place to build actual skills. Whether it's mastering a new language, improving your writing, or learning to play an instrument, these pursuits require time and dedication—things you'll have in spades once you quit social media.

Here's a challenge: pick a skill you've always wanted to learn and dedicate the time you would have spent on social media to it. Watch how quickly you improve. The results might surprise you.

A New Sense Of Control

Quitting social media gives you back control over your life. You're no longer a puppet to the whims of algorithms and digital trends. Instead, you're the master of your time and focus.

You get to decide how you spend your hours, what you work on, and how you live your life. It's a refreshing change from being constantly pulled in a hundred different directions by notifications and updates.

The Ultimate Reward: Personal Fulfillment

In the end, the real reward of quitting social media is personal fulfillment. It's finding satisfaction in your accomplishments, joy in your experiences, and contentment in your relationships. It's about living a life that's not defined by digital metrics but by real, tangible moments of happiness and success.

So, here's to reclaiming your time, rediscovering your focus, and enjoying the genuine experiences life has to offer. You've taken the first step by stepping away from social media. Now, make the most of it.

Next we are going to dive into practical steps for quitting social media and how to make the transition as smooth as possible. It's time to turn those grand ideas into action.

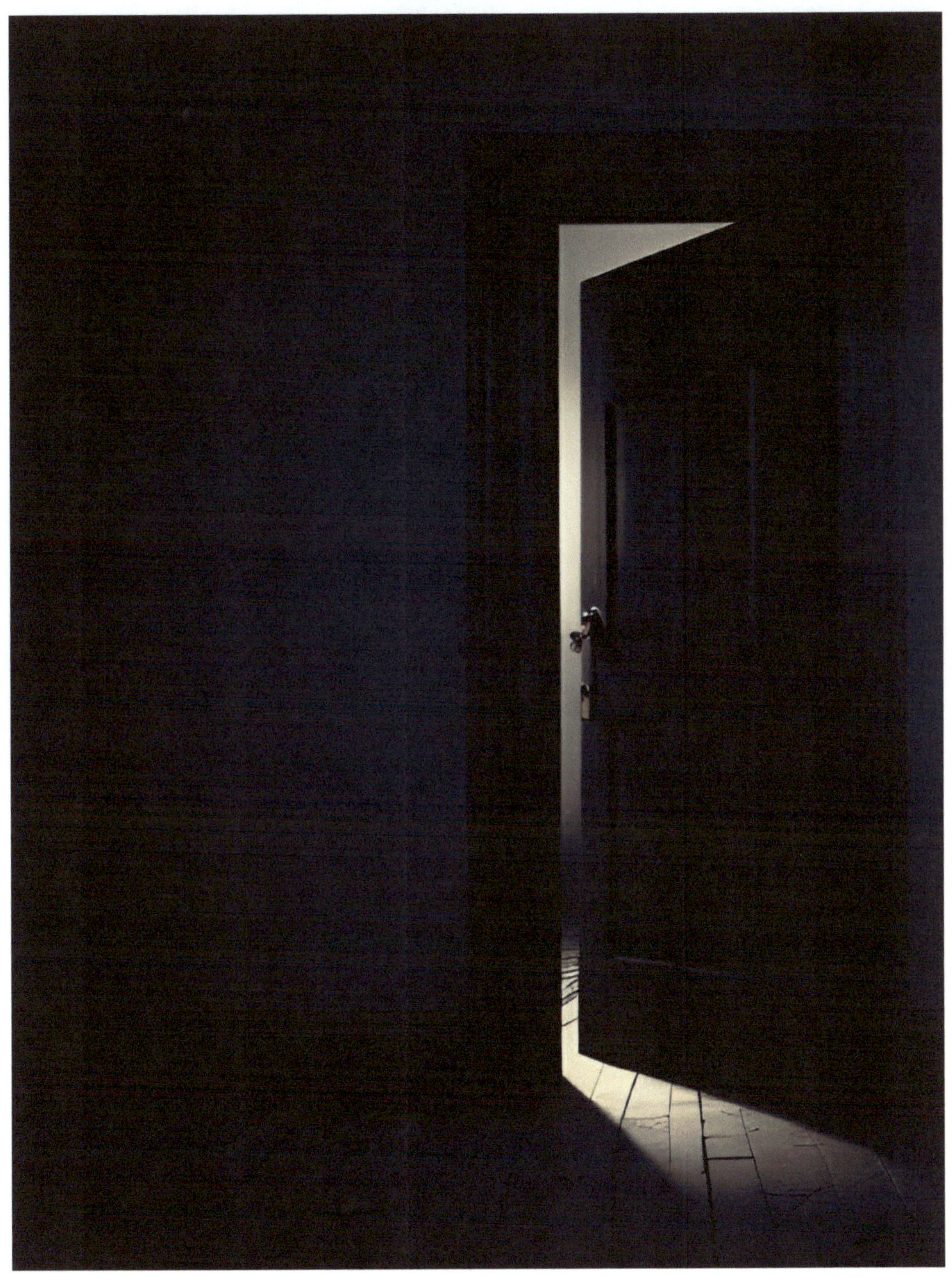

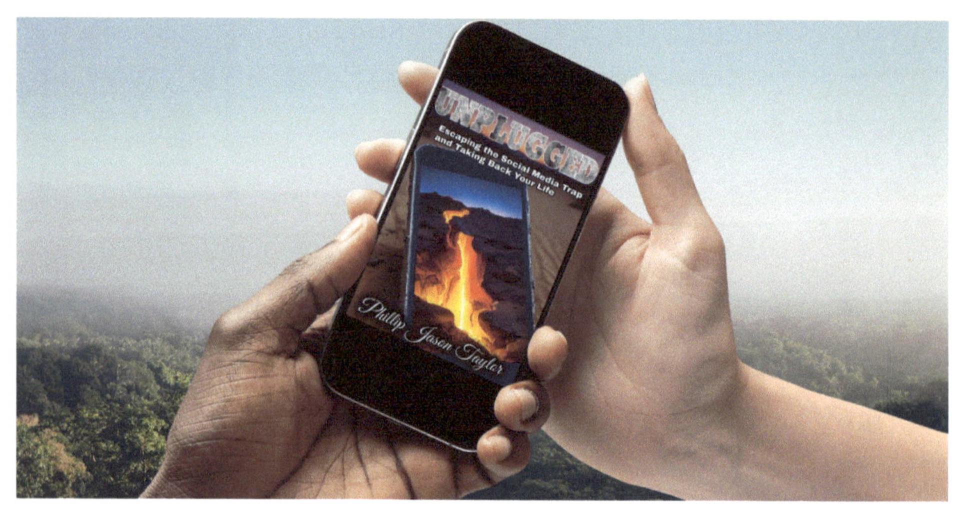

THE HOW-TO GUIDE FOR QUITTING SOCIAL MEDIA

Step 1: The Great Deactivation

Alright, you've decided to quit social media—now what? First things first: it's time for the big step, the digital equivalent of a dramatic breakup. Deactivate your accounts. Don't just log off; make it official. Most platforms offer an option to deactivate or delete your account. And let's face it, if you're not going to be checking back, why not just take the plunge?

But before you go all scorched earth, make sure you've saved any important data. Download your photos, messages, and any content you might actually want to keep. Once you're deactivated, there's no turning back (or at least it's a lot more difficult).

Step 2: Set Up Your Digital Detox Plan

You wouldn't quit a job without a plan, so don't quit social media without one either. Here's what to include in your detox plan:

- Identify Your Triggers: What's the first thing you'll do when you feel the urge to check your social media? Maybe it's a new hobby, a workout, or even a good book. Knowing your triggers helps you stay on track.

- Create New Routines: Fill the time you would have spent scrolling with something productive or enjoyable. This could be a daily walk, learning a new skill, or catching up on that Netflix series you've been ignoring.

- Inform Your Contacts: Let your friends and family know that you're taking a break from social media. This will help them understand why you're not responding to messages or liking their posts. Plus, it'll save you from awkward questions.

Step 3: Find Your New Source Of Entertainment

So, what do you do with all this extra time? Start by exploring new interests and hobbies. Remember those things you used to enjoy before social media took over? Revisit them! Here are a few ideas:

- Read More: Whether it's fiction, non-fiction, or that self-help book you bought on a whim, immerse yourself in the world of books.

- Get Creative: Start a new art project, learn to play an instrument, or try your hand at writing. Your creativity won't know what hit it.

- Exercise: Physical activity is a great way to spend time and improve your health. Plus, you can enjoy the endorphins without needing a like button to validate your workout.

Step 4: Reconnect With The Real World

Now that you've freed yourself from the digital noise, it's time to re-engage with the world around you. This means:

- Face-to-Face Interaction: Spend more time with friends and family in person. Engage in meaningful conversations and create real memories.
- Community Involvement: Get involved in local events or volunteer opportunities. It's a great way to meet new people and make a positive impact in your community.
- Mindfulness: Practice being present in the moment. Enjoy your surroundings, savor your meals, and engage fully with your experiences.

Step 5: Embrace The Digital Minimalism

The goal here isn't just to quit social media; it's to embrace a more intentional digital life. This means:

- Curate Your Online Presence: If you must use social media for professional reasons, keep it minimal and purposeful. Avoid the endless scrolling and focus on content that adds value.
- Set Boundaries: Limit your screen time and establish rules for when and how you use your devices. For example, no screens during meals or before bedtime.
- Be Selective with Apps: Choose apps and digital tools that genuinely enhance your life and avoid those that are just time sinks.

Step 6: Reflect And Adjust

After your initial detox period, take some time to reflect on how you're feeling. Ask yourself:

- Am I more relaxed? If so, how can I keep this feeling going?

- Do I miss anything about social media? If so, what can I do to address those needs in a healthier way?
- What have I gained? Celebrate the positive changes and continue to nurture them.

If you find certain aspects of social media beneficial, consider reintroducing them in a controlled and mindful manner. The goal isn't to completely cut yourself off but to strike a balance that works for you.

Step 7: Celebrate Your Success

You've made it this far—give yourself a pat on the back! Embracing a life without social media is a significant achievement. Celebrate your success by treating yourself to something special, whether it's a day out, a new book, or simply enjoying a quiet evening at home.

Remember, quitting social media isn't about deprivation; it's about rediscovering the joy of real-life experiences and connections. Enjoy the freedom, relish in your new-found time, and keep making choices that enhance your well-being.

In the next chapter, we'll delve into how to maintain your new lifestyle and avoid falling back into old habits. Stay tuned for more on living a fulfilling life without the social media shackles.

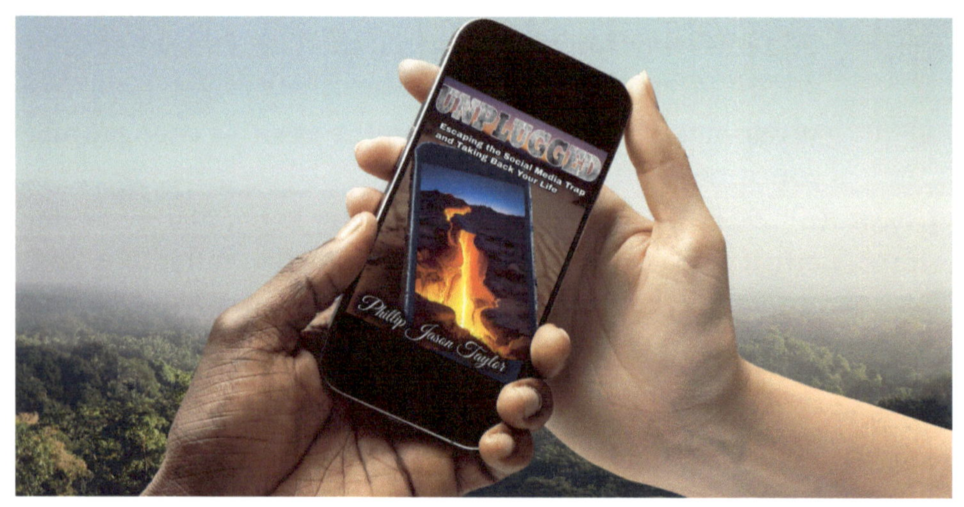

MAINTAINING YOUR NEW LIFESTYLE AND AVOIDING RELAPSE

The Temptation Trap: Staying Strong

Congratulations on making it this far—you're officially free from the social media vortex! But before you start patting yourself on the back too hard, let's address the inevitable temptation to slip back into old habits. After all, breaking a habit is one thing; staying broken is another.

Here's the deal: social media is designed to be addictive. It's not just a platform; it's a carefully engineered machine that preys on your need for validation and distraction. So, how do you avoid falling back into the trap?

First, acknowledge that the temptation will come. You'll get the itch to check what's going on, to see who's posted what, or to scroll through your feed just because you're bored. Recognize these moments as they happen and remind yourself why you decided to quit in the first place.

Create New, Healthy Habits

Replacing an old habit with a new one is one of the best ways to ensure you don't fall back into your old ways. If social media was your go-to for boredom, you need a new outlet. Here are some suggestions to fill the void:

- Explore New Hobbies: Dive into activities you've always wanted to try but never had the time for. Whether it's gardening, woodworking, or bird-watching, find something that excites you.
- Socialize in Person: Make a conscious effort to engage in face-to-face interactions. Organize meetups, join clubs, or attend events where you can connect with people in the real world.
- Practice Mindfulness: Incorporate mindfulness practices into your daily routine. Meditation, journaling, or simply spending quiet time alone can help you stay centered and reduce the urge to check your phone.

Set Boundaries For Technology Use

If you can't entirely cut out technology, set boundaries to keep it from interfering with your life. Consider:

- Screen-Free Zones: Designate certain areas of your home as screen-free zones to encourage more offline activities. For instance, keep your bedroom a tech-free sanctuary.
- Scheduled Tech Time: Allocate specific times of the day for checking emails or using apps. By setting limits, you prevent technology from consuming your entire day.

- Device-Free Meals: Make meals a tech-free experience. Use this time to connect with others or simply enjoy your food without distractions.

Find A Support System

Breaking away from social media is easier when you have support. Surround yourself with people who respect your decision and who can help you stay accountable. Share your goals with friends and family and let them know how they can support you.

Consider finding or creating a community of like-minded individuals who are also taking a break from social media. This can be a great way to share experiences, offer mutual encouragement, and avoid feeling isolated.

Reflect On Your Progress

Regularly take time to reflect on your journey and assess how your life has changed since quitting social media. Ask yourself:

- What positive changes have I noticed? Focus on the improvements in your well-being, productivity, and relationships.
- What challenges have I faced? Identify any difficulties you've encountered and strategize on how to overcome them.
- How can I continue to grow? Set new personal goals or pursue new interests to keep yourself engaged and motivated.

Handling Social Media Cravings

Even after significant time away, cravings can strike. When they do:

- Identify Triggers: Recognize what triggers your craving and address it directly. Is it boredom, stress, or curiosity? Find healthy ways to manage these triggers.
- Distract Yourself: Engage in a new activity or hobby to divert your attention. Read a book, go for a walk, or try a new craft.
- Remind Yourself of Your Reasons: Revisit the reasons you decided to quit social media. Reflect on the benefits you've experienced and the goals you've achieved.

Embrace The New Normal

Adapting to a life without social media is a process. Embrace it as your new normal rather than a temporary change. The longer you live without it, the more natural it will feel. Celebrate your successes and continue to nurture the habits that support your well-being.

Remember, quitting social media doesn't mean you're missing out on life; it means you're choosing to engage with it more deeply. By maintaining your new lifestyle, you're investing in a more fulfilling and balanced existence.

In the next chapter, we'll wrap up with a final look at the benefits of living a social media-free life and how to keep the positive momentum going.

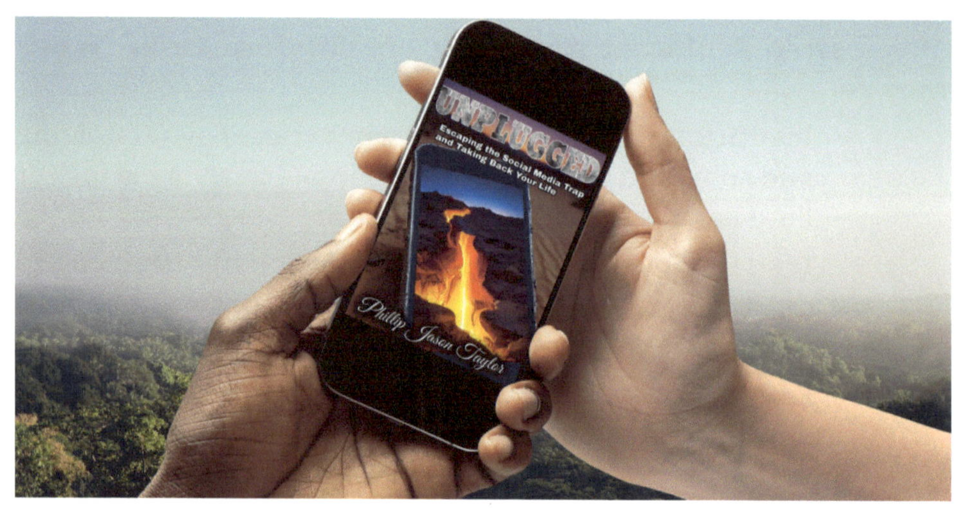

EMBRACING THE SOCIAL MEDIA-FREE LIFE: THE FINAL WORD

The Benefits You've Gained

By now, you've had a chance to experience the many benefits of living without social media. Let's take a moment to bask in these advantages and appreciate how far you've come:

- Increased Productivity: Without the constant pull of notifications, you've probably noticed a boost in your ability to focus and get things done. Whether it's work, hobbies, or personal projects, your productivity has likely soared.

- Improved Mental Health: Social media can be a breeding ground for stress, anxiety, and comparison. Without it, you've likely experienced a decrease in these negative emotions and an increase in overall well-being.

- Deeper Connections: You've probably found that your relationships are more meaningful and fulfilling. Engaging with people face-to-face and in real life has deepened your connections and made them more genuine.

- Rediscovered Interests: You've had the opportunity to explore new hobbies and passions. From creative pursuits to physical activities, you've reconnected with interests that bring joy and fulfillment.

Maintaining Your New Lifestyle

Maintaining a social media-free lifestyle requires ongoing effort and commitment. Here are some tips to keep the positive momentum going:

- Regular Check-Ins: Periodically assess how you're feeling and what you've accomplished. Celebrate your successes and adjust your strategies if necessary.

- Set New Goals: Keep challenging yourself by setting new personal goals and pursuing interests that excite you. This keeps you motivated and engaged in your new lifestyle.

- Stay Mindful: Continue practicing mindfulness and being present in your daily life. This helps you stay grounded and focused on what truly matters.

The Joy Of Authentic Living

Living without social media offers a unique opportunity to experience life in its most authentic form. You're not caught up in the digital noise or the pressures of online validation. Instead, you're free to:

- Enjoy the Moment: Appreciate the small, everyday moments that often go unnoticed when you're absorbed in your feed. Whether it's a beautiful sunset or a heartfelt conversation, savor these experiences.

- Pursue Genuine Happiness: Seek out activities and relationships that bring you real joy and satisfaction. Your happiness isn't dictated by likes or comments but by the meaningful experiences you create for yourself.

Navigating Social Media If Necessary

If you find that social media is necessary for certain aspects of your life—such as professional networking or staying in touch with distant friends—approach it with intention:

- Use It Wisely: Limit your use to specific tasks or times of day. Avoid falling back into old habits by setting clear boundaries.

- Be Selective: Choose platforms and interactions that add value to your life. Avoid getting caught up in the endless scroll or the pressure to be constantly engaged.

- Regular Detoxes: Consider periodic breaks from social media to refresh and recalibrate. This helps maintain a healthy balance and keeps you grounded.

Final Thoughts

Congratulations on completing this journey to a social media-free life! Embracing this lifestyle is not just about quitting a habit; it's about choosing a more fulfilling, authentic way of living. You've made a powerful choice to prioritize your well-being and invest in real-life experiences.

Remember, the freedom you've gained is a valuable asset. Continue to nurture it by staying mindful, setting new goals, and embracing the joys of authentic living. Your life is now richer, more focused, and filled with possibilities.

As you move forward, carry with you the lessons learned and the benefits gained from this experience. Celebrate your success and enjoy the positive changes that come from living a life not dictated by digital distractions.

Here's to a future where you live fully, engage deeply, and cherish every moment. Cheers to your social media-free life!

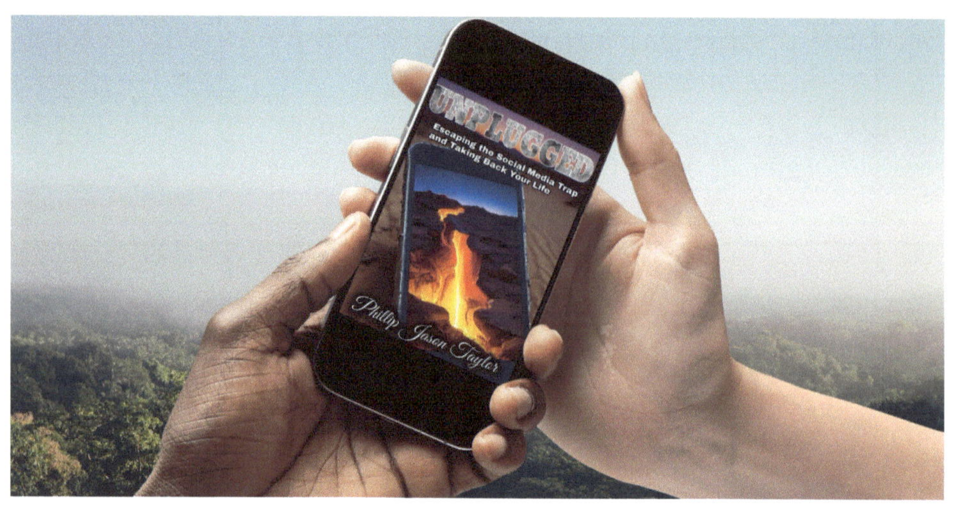

TOOLS AND APPS FOR MANAGING DIGITAL HABITS

1. Time Management

- RescueTime: Tracks your computer and smartphone usage to give you insights into where your time goes. Helps identify time sinks and set goals for better productivity.

- Toggl: A simple time-tracking tool that helps you understand how you spend your time and can improve your productivity.

- Focus@Will: Provides music designed to enhance focus and productivity. Perfect for creating a distraction-free work environment.

2. Mindfulness and Well-Being

- Headspace: Offers guided meditation and mindfulness exercises to help reduce stress and improve mental clarity.

- Calm: Provides meditation, sleep stories, and relaxation

techniques to support overall mental health and well-being.

- Insight Timer: Features a wide range of free meditation sessions and mindfulness practices.

3. Digital Detox

- Forest: Helps you stay focused by growing a virtual tree that flourishes as long as you don't use your phone. Great for reducing phone distractions.

- Freedom: Blocks distracting websites and apps across all your devices, allowing you to stay focused on your work.

- Stay Focused: A browser extension that limits time spent on distracting websites.

4. Productivity

- Todoist: A task management app that helps you organize and prioritize your tasks and projects effectively.

- Notion: An all-in-one workspace for notes, tasks, databases, and collaboration. Helps streamline your workflow and stay organized.

- Evernote: A note-taking app that helps you capture and organize your ideas, tasks, and documents.

5. Goal Setting and Habit Tracking

- Habitica: Turns goal-setting and habit-building into a game, making it fun to develop new habits and track progress.

- Streaks: Helps you build good habits by tracking your progress and encouraging you to maintain streaks of consecutive days.

- Coach.me: Offers habit tracking and personal coaching to help you achieve your goals and build positive habits.

6. Digital Wellness

- Screen Time (iOS): Built into iOS, it helps monitor and manage screen time on Apple devices, allowing you to set limits and track usage.

- Digital Wellbeing: A suite of tools by Google for Android devices that helps you understand and control your screen time.

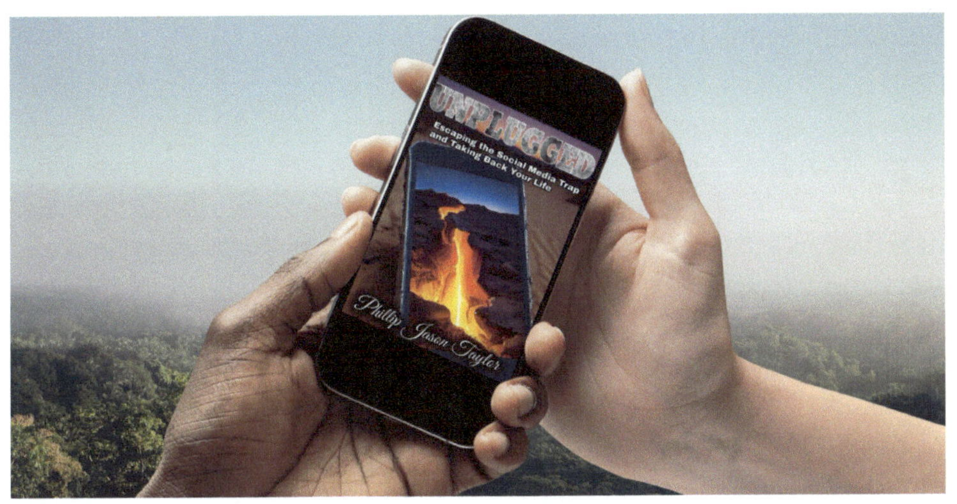

AUTHOR'S NOTE

In writing this book, I've drawn from my own experiences with social media—an area of my life that's been as tumultuous as it has been enlightening. I've faced the dark side of social media first-hand: group bullying that left me questioning my self-worth, the temptation to overshare personal details that compromised my privacy, and even employment issues that arose from my online presence.

Social media, for me, was a double-edged sword. On one hand, it offered a platform for self-expression and connection. On the other, it became a breeding ground for negativity and unintended consequences. I've been on the receiving end of group bullying— a harsh reminder of how digital anonymity can sometimes bring out the worst in people. The sting of cruel comments and the weight of collective judgment was a painful lesson in the pitfalls of online interactions.

I also found myself caught in the trap of oversharing, thinking that sharing more of my personal life would bring me closer to others. Instead, it often led to unwanted scrutiny and a loss of privacy. It became apparent that the more I revealed, the more vulnerable I became to judgment and exploitation.

Perhaps most unsettling were the employment issues that arose from my social media activity. My online presence, once a source of professional pride, became a liability. I found that my digital footprint had a way of following me into professional spaces, affecting opportunities and relationships in ways I hadn't anticipated.

These challenges were instrumental in guiding me towards a social media-free lifestyle. They taught me the importance of protecting my mental health, preserving my privacy, and managing my online persona with intention and care. My journey from social media reliance to reclaiming my peace has been a transformative one, and I share it with you not as a perfect solution, but as a heartfelt exploration of what it means to live authentically in the digital age.

If you've struggled with similar issues, know that you're not alone. The path to a more balanced and fulfilling life is one of self-discovery and courage. I hope that my experiences and the strategies outlined in this book will offer you insight and encouragement as you navigate your own journey towards a healthier relationship with social media.

Thank you for joining me on this path. May you find the freedom and fulfillment that I have found in living beyond the digital noise.

Warm regards,

Phillip Jason Taylor

Readers are always welcome to share their honest thoughts about this book. Reviews are entirely voluntary and greatly help others decide whether this book is right for them.

Leave your review of "Unplugged"

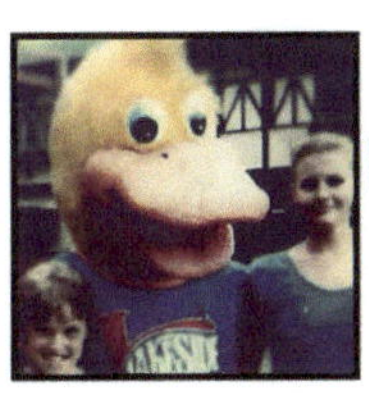

Phillip Dedicates this book to his hero, his mother, local wonder Woman
Beverly Taylor

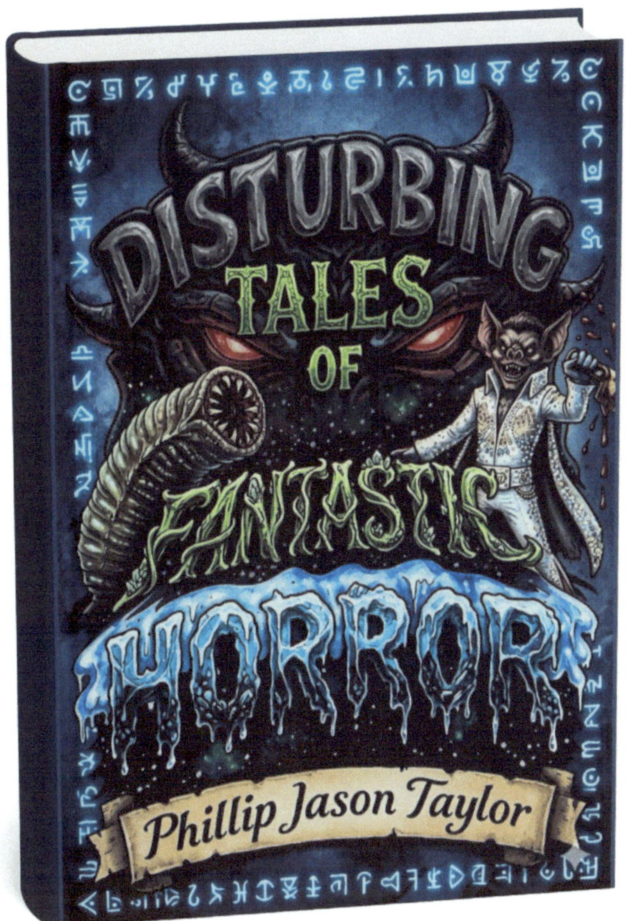

Learn More About Phillip

BOOKS BY THIS AUTHOR

How To Be The Best Nurse For The Public

Howdy, partner! Ready to rustle up some top-notch nursing skills? How to Be the Best Nurse for the Public is your guide to blending compassionate care with a hearty dose of frontier spirit. Whether you're tending to a bustling town or a quiet prairie, this book'll show ya how to saddle up and deliver healthcare that's as warm as a campfire and as reliable as a trusty steed.

In these pages, you'll find:

Straight-shootin' tips for top-tier patient care, delivered with a friendly, down-to-earth approach.
Ranch-tested strategies for handling high-stress situations with calm and confidence.
Wisdom from the Wild West to guide you in creating connections and providing comfort to every patient.
So, grab your hat and get ready to ride into the world of nursing. This guide will help you become a healthcare hero, no matter where your practice takes you.

Terrifying Tales From The Dark: Nightmares You Can't Wake From

Inside, you'll encounter:

Cursed towns and haunted rooms where time itself turns against you.

Ordinary people who make one mistake… and pay for it in ways they can't imagine.

Dark entities that don't lurk under the bed — they live inside your mind.

Nightmares so vivid they feel like memories when you wake.

Enter the shadows — where every sound has meaning, every silence has weight, and sleep offers no escape.
Terrifying Tales from the Darkis a collection of short horror stories that crawl beneath your skin and stay there.
These are the dreams you can't shake. The whispers behind the walls. The truths you wish weren't real.
Beautifully written, deeply unsettling, and impossible to forget, Terrifying Tales from the Dark is a collection for readers who crave the thrill of being afraid — and the art of horror.
DARE TO READ IN THE DARK